QUIT CRAVINGS FOR SUGAR AND WELCOME TO A HEALTHIER YOU WITH THE BLOOD SUGAR SOLUTION

Darryl S. Johnson

Table of Content

Introduction

The world we live in today is fast-paced, full of stress, and inundated with unhealthy food choices that can have a significant impact on our health, particularly our blood sugar levels. High blood sugar levels can cause a range of health problems, including diabetes, heart disease, and stroke, to name a few. If left uncontrolled, it can have a detrimental effect on our overall well-being.

But what if we told you that there is a solution to managing your blood sugar levels and regaining your health? Welcome to "The Blood Sugar Solution."

In this book, you will discover the latest scientific research and cutting-edge techniques for managing your blood sugar levels, preventing and reversing diabetes, and achieving optimal health. You will learn how to create a personalized plan that is tailored to your unique needs, preferences, and lifestyle.

This book is not just another diet book or quick fix solution. It is a comprehensive guide that takes a holistic approach to managing blood sugar levels, covering everything from nutrition and exercise to stress management and sleep. The strategies outlined in this book are sustainable, practical, and easy to implement, making it accessible for anyone looking to improve their health and well-being.

Whether you are someone who has been struggling with high blood sugar levels for years, or simply looking to optimize your health and prevent future health issues, "The Blood Sugar Solution" has something for you. Get ready to take control of your health, achieve balanced blood sugar levels, and live your best life yet.

Chapter 1

Understanding Blood Sugar

Blood sugar, also known as glucose, is a type of sugar that serves as the primary source of energy for the body's cells. It is obtained from the foods we eat, particularly carbohydrates, and is transported throughout the body via the bloodstream. In a healthy individual, blood sugar levels are regulated tightly to ensure that they remain within a narrow range.

The Importance of Balanced Blood Sugar Levels

Maintaining balanced blood sugar levels is crucial for overall health and well-being. High blood sugar levels, known as hyperglycemia, can lead to a range of health problems, including diabetes, heart disease, and stroke. Symptoms of hyperglycemia may include increased thirst, frequent urination, fatigue, blurred vision, and slow healing of cuts and wounds.

On the other hand, low blood sugar levels, known as hypoglycemia, can cause symptoms such as shakiness, dizziness, sweating, confusion, and even loss of consciousness. Prolonged or severe hypoglycemia can be dangerous and even life-threatening.

Factors That Affect Blood Sugar Levels

Blood sugar levels can be affected by a variety of factors, including diet, exercise, stress, medications, and health conditions. Consuming foods high in sugar or refined carbohydrates, for example, can cause a rapid increase in blood sugar levels, whereas consuming high-fiber foods or foods containing healthy fats and proteins can help to stabilize blood sugar levels.

Exercise can also have a significant impact on blood sugar levels. Physical activity helps to increase insulin sensitivity, allowing the body to use insulin more effectively to transport glucose into the cells. This can help to lower blood sugar levels and reduce the risk of developing type 2 diabetes.

Stress is another factor that can affect blood sugar levels. When we are under stress, our bodies release hormones such as cortisol and adrenaline, which can cause blood sugar levels to rise. Over time, chronic stress can lead to insulin resistance, a condition in which the body becomes less responsive to insulin and less able to regulate blood sugar levels effectively. Blood sugar, also known as glucose, is a type of sugar that is found in the bloodstream. It is the primary source of energy for the body's cells and is essential for normal bodily functions.

The Role of Insulin in Blood Sugar Regulation

Insulin is a hormone produced by the pancreas that plays a crucial role in blood sugar regulation. When blood sugar levels rise after a meal, insulin is released into the bloodstream to signal the body's cells to absorb glucose from the blood and use it for energy. Insulin helps to maintain blood sugar levels within a normal range, preventing them from getting too high (hyperglycemia) or too low (hypoglycemia).

The Importance of Blood Sugar Control

Maintaining healthy blood sugar levels is crucial for overall health and wellbeing. Elevated blood sugar levels can lead to a range of health problems, including:

1.Diabetes: Diabetes is a chronic condition in which the body is unable to produce or effectively use insulin, leading to elevated blood sugar levels. If left untreated, diabetes can lead to a range of complications, including heart disease, nerve damage, and kidney damage.

2.Heart disease: Elevated blood sugar levels can damage blood vessels and increase the risk of heart disease.

3.Nerve damage: High blood sugar levels can damage nerves, leading to numbness, tingling, and other sensations.

4.Eye damage: Elevated blood sugar levels can damage blood vessels in the eyes, leading to vision problems.

5.Kidney damage: High blood sugar levels can damage the kidneys, leading to kidney disease.

Strategies for Blood Sugar Management

There are several strategies for managing blood sugar levels, including:

1.Diet: A healthy diet that is rich in whole foods, fruits, and vegetables and low in processed foods and added sugars can help to regulate blood sugar levels.

2.Exercise: Regular exercise can help to improve insulin sensitivity and lower blood sugar levels.

3.Medication: Medications, such as insulin and oral hypoglycemic agents, can help to regulate blood sugar levels in people with diabetes.

4.Blood sugar monitoring: Regular monitoring of blood sugar levels can help to identify fluctuations and allow for timely interventions.

Conclusion

Blood sugar regulation is crucial for overall health and wellbeing, and elevated blood sugar levels can lead to a range of health problems. By understanding the role of insulin in blood sugar regulation and implementing effective strategies for blood sugar management, individuals can improve their health and prevent complications associated with diabetes. In the following chapters, we will explore these strategies in more detail and provide practical tips and expert advice for managing blood sugar levels.

Chapter 2

The Role of Nutrition

Nutrition plays a crucial role in managing blood sugar levels. The foods we eat provide the glucose that our bodies use as energy, but not all foods are created equal when it comes to their impact on blood sugar levels. Understanding the glycemic index and glycemic load can help individuals make healthy food choices and create a balanced diet that supports healthy blood sugar levels.

The Glycemic Index and Glycemic Load

The glycemic index (GI) is a measure of how quickly foods raise blood sugar levels. Foods with a high GI, such as white bread, white rice, and sugary drinks, cause a rapid increase in blood sugar levels, whereas foods with a low GI, such as vegetables, fruits, and whole grains, cause a slower and more gradual increase in blood sugar levels.

The glycemic load (GL) takes into account both the quality and quantity of carbohydrates in a food, as well as the fiber and fat content. Foods with a high GL, such as potatoes and white rice, can cause a rapid increase in blood sugar levels even if their GI is relatively low. On the other hand, foods with a low GL, such as beans and lentils, can provide a sustained source of energy without causing a rapid increase in blood sugar levels.

Healthy Food Choices for Managing Blood Sugar Levels

Making healthy food choices is essential for managing blood sugar levels and preventing health problems related to imbalanced blood sugar. Some of the key foods to include in a healthy diet for blood sugar management include:

i.Non-starchy vegetables: These include leafy greens, broccoli, cauliflower, peppers, and more. These are low in calories and carbohydrates, and high in fiber and other important nutrients.

ii.Whole grains: Whole grain foods such as quinoa, brown rice, and whole wheat bread are good sources of fiber and other nutrients that help to slow down the absorption of glucose.

iii.Lean proteins: Protein sources such as chicken, fish, tofu, and beans can help to slow down the absorption of glucose and provide a sustained source of energy.

iv.Healthy fats: Healthy fats such as olive oil, avocado, nuts, and seeds can help to improve insulin sensitivity and support healthy blood sugar levels.

The Impact of Carbohydrate Quality on Blood Sugar

In addition to the GI and GL, the quality of carbohydrates consumed can also impact blood sugar levels. Simple carbohydrates (such as refined sugar and white bread) are rapidly absorbed into the bloodstream, causing a rapid rise in blood sugar levels. Complex carbohydrates (such as whole grains and vegetables) are digested more slowly, leading to a more gradual rise in blood sugar levels.

Strategies for Managing Carbohydrate Intake

Carbohydrates are an important source of energy for the body, but the type and amount consumed can have a significant impact on blood sugar levels. By understanding the impact of carbohydrates on blood sugar and implementing effective strategies for managing carbohydrate intake, individuals can improve their blood sugar control and overall health.

Managing carbohydrate intake is an important strategy for regulating blood sugar levels. Some effective strategies include:

1.Choosing low GI and GL carbohydrates: Consuming carbohydrates with a low GI and GL can help to regulate blood sugar levels and prevent spikes.

2.Balancing carbohydrates with protein and fat: Combining carbohydrates with protein and fat can slow down the absorption of carbohydrates and prevent rapid spikes in blood sugar levels.

3.Portion control: Controlling portion sizes can help to limit the amount of carbohydrates consumed and prevent spikes in blood sugar levels.

4.Timing of carbohydrate consumption: Consuming carbohydrates at the right times (such as before or after exercise) can help to regulate blood sugar levels

Conclusion

In conclusion, nutrition plays a crucial role in managing blood sugar levels. Understanding the glycemic index and glycemic load can help individuals make healthy food choices and create a balanced diet that supports healthy blood sugar levels. By including a variety of non-starchy vegetables, whole grains, lean proteins, and healthy fats in their diet, individuals can help to maintain balanced blood sugar levels and achieve optimal health. In the following chapters, we have explore additional strategies for managing blood sugar levels, including the importance of exercise, stress management, and sleep, more detail and provide practical tips and expert advice for managing carbohydrate intake.

Chapter 3

Exercise and Blood Sugar Management

Exercise is a powerful tool for managing blood sugar levels and improving overall health. Regular physical activity helps to increase insulin sensitivity, allowing the body to use insulin more effectively to transport glucose into the cells. This can help to lower blood sugar levels and reduce the risk of developing type 2 diabetes.

The Role of Protein and Fat in Blood Sugar Control

While carbohydrates are the primary source of energy for the body, protein and fat also play important roles in blood sugar control. In this chapter, we will explore the role of protein and fat in blood sugar regulation and provide tips for incorporating these macronutrients into a healthy diet.

Protein and Blood Sugar Control

Protein is an essential macronutrient that plays a key role in a variety of bodily functions. When protein is consumed, it is broken down into amino acids, which are used to build and repair tissues, synthesize hormones and enzymes, and support immune function.

Protein also has a minimal impact on blood sugar levels. Unlike carbohydrates, which are rapidly absorbed into the bloodstream and cause blood sugar spikes, protein is digested slowly and does not cause significant fluctuations in blood sugar levels.

In addition to its impact on blood sugar control, protein is also important for satiety and weight management. Consuming adequate amounts of protein can help to reduce appetite, increase feelings of fullness, and support healthy weight management.

Sources of protein include:

i.Lean meats and poultry
ii.Fish and seafood
iii.Eggs
iv.Beans and legumes
v.Nuts and seeds
vi.Dairy products
vii.Fat and Blood Sugar Control

Fat is another macronutrient that plays an important role in blood sugar control. Like protein, fat is digested slowly and does not cause significant fluctuations in blood sugar levels.

In addition to its impact on blood sugar control, fat is important for a variety of bodily functions. It is used to produce hormones and support the absorption of fat-soluble vitamins (such as vitamins A, D, E, and K). Fat is also important for satiety and can help to reduce appetite and increase feelings of fullness.

However, not all fats are created equal. Consuming too much saturated and trans fats (found in foods such as red meat, butter, and fried foods) can increase the risk of heart disease and other health problems. Instead, individuals should focus on consuming healthy fats, such as monounsaturated and polyunsaturated fats (found in foods such as nuts, seeds, avocados, and fatty fish).

Incorporating Protein and Fat into a Healthy Diet

Incorporating protein and fat into a healthy diet can help to regulate blood sugar levels, support satiety, and provide a range of important nutrients. Some strategies for incorporating protein and fat into a healthy diet include:

Choosing lean sources of protein, such as chicken, fish, and legumes

Incorporating healthy fats, such as nuts, seeds, and avocados, into meals and snacks

Balancing meals with a combination of protein, carbohydrates, and healthy fats

Choosing cooking methods that minimize the use of added fats (such as baking, broiling, or grilling)

The Benefits of Exercise for Blood Sugar Management

In addition to improving insulin sensitivity, exercise offers a range of other benefits for blood sugar management and overall health. These include:

1.Improved glucose control: Regular exercise can help to lower blood sugar levels and improve glucose control, even in individuals with diabetes.

2.Increased energy expenditure: Exercise burns calories and helps to maintain a healthy weight, which is important for blood sugar management.

3.Reduced insulin resistance: Exercise helps to improve insulin sensitivity, reducing the risk of developing insulin resistance and type 2 diabetes.

4.Loweredinflammation: Chronic inflammation is associated with insulin resistance and other health problems. Exercise helps to reduce inflammation and support overall health.

5.Improved cardiovascular health: Regular exercise can help to lower blood pressure, improve cholesterol levels, and reduce the risk of heart disease and stroke.

Types of Exercise for Blood Sugar Management

There are many different types of exercise that can be effective for managing blood sugar levels. Some of the most effective types of exercise include:

1.Aerobic exercise: Activities such as brisk walking, jogging, cycling, and swimming can help to improve cardiovascular health and lower blood sugar levels.

2.Resistance training: Strength training exercises such as weight lifting can help to build muscle mass and improve insulin sensitivity.

3.High-intensity interval training (HIIT): HIIT involves short bursts of intense exercise followed by periods of rest. This type of exercise can be effective for improving glucose control and insulin sensitivity.

4.Yoga: Yoga can help to reduce stress and improve flexibility, which can support healthy blood sugar levels.

Exercise and Blood Sugar Management Tips

To get the most benefit from exercise for blood sugar management, it is important to make it a regular part of your routine. Some tips for incorporating exercise into your routine include:

i.Start slowly: If you are new to exercise or have not exercised in a while, start with low-intensity activities such as walking or gentle yoga.

ii.Set realistic goals: Set goals that are achievable and realistic for your fitness level and schedule.

iii.Make it enjoyable: Choose activities that you enjoy and that fit into your lifestyle.

iv.Monitor blood sugar levels: Monitor your blood sugar levels before, during, and after exercise to determine how it affects your levels.

v.Stay hydrated: Drink plenty of water before, during, and after exercise to stay hydrated.

Conclusion

In conclusion, exercise is a powerful tool for managing blood sugar levels and improving overall health. Regular physical activity can help to increase insulin sensitivity, improve glucose control, and reduce the risk of developing type 2 diabetes. By incorporating a variety of aerobic, resistance, and flexibility exercises into their routine, individuals can help to maintain healthy blood sugar levels and achieve optimal health. In the following chapters, we will explore additional strategies for managing blood sugar levels, including stress management and sleep.

Chapter 4:

Exercise and Blood Sugar Management

Exercise is an important component of a healthy lifestyle and can play a significant role in blood sugar management. Regular exercise has been shown to improve insulin sensitivity, reduce blood sugar levels, and reduce the risk of developing type 2 diabetes.

The Benefits of Exercise for Blood Sugar Management

Regular exercise offers a range of benefits for blood sugar management, including:

1.Improved insulin sensitivity: Exercise helps the body to use insulin more effectively to transport glucose into the cells, improving insulin sensitivity and blood sugar control.

2.Reduced blood sugar levels: Exercise can help to reduce blood sugar levels by increasing glucose uptake by the muscles and improving insulin sensitivity.

3.Weight management: Exercise helps to burn calories and maintain a healthy weight, reducing the risk of developing type 2 diabetes.

4.Lowered risk of complications: Regular exercise can help to reduce the risk of developing complications associated with diabetes, including heart disease and nerve damage.

Types of Exercise for Blood Sugar Management

Different types of exercise can offer different benefits for blood sugar management. Some types of exercise that may be particularly beneficial for blood sugar control include:

1.Aerobic exercise: This type of exercise, such as jogging or cycling, helps to improve cardiovascular health, burn calories, and improve insulin sensitivity.

2.Resistance training: Resistance training, such as weight lifting, can help to build muscle mass and improve insulin sensitivity.

3.High-intensity interval training (HIIT): HIIT involves short bursts of intense exercise followed by periods of rest. This type of exercise has been shown to improve insulin sensitivity and blood sugar control.

4.Yoga: Yoga can help to reduce stress levels and improve insulin sensitivity, making it a useful tool for blood sugar management.

Exercise Safety and Precautions

While exercise can offer significant benefits for blood sugar management, it is important to take appropriate precautions to avoid injury or adverse effects. Some tips for exercising safely with diabetes include:

1.Consult with a healthcare provider before starting an exercise program.

2.Monitor blood sugar levels before, during, and after exercise to avoid hypoglycemia (low blood sugar) or hyperglycemia (high blood sugar).

3.Carry a source of fast-acting carbohydrates, such as glucose tablets or a sports drink, to treat hypoglycemia.

4.Wear appropriate footwear and clothing and avoid exercising in extreme temperatures.

5.Take appropriate precautions to avoid foot injuries, as people with diabetes may have reduced circulation or nerve damage.

Conclusion

Exercise is an important tool for blood sugar management and overall health. Regular exercise can improve insulin sensitivity, reduce blood sugar levels, and reduce the risk of developing complications associated with diabetes. Different types of exercise can offer different benefits, and it is important to take appropriate precautions to avoid injury or adverse effects. By consulting with a healthcare provider, monitoring blood sugar levels, and taking appropriate safety measures, individuals with diabetes can safely and effectively incorporate exercise into their routine. In the following chapters, we will explore additional strategies for managing blood sugar levels, including nutrition and medication.

Chapter 5

Sleep and Blood Sugar Management

Getting enough quality sleep is essential for overall health and can play a significant role in blood sugar management. Sleep deprivation and poor sleep quality have been linked to insulin resistance, weight gain, and an increased risk of developing type 2 diabetes.

Stress is a common and often unavoidable part of daily life. While some stress can be beneficial and help to motivate and energize us, chronic or excessive stress can have negative effects on our health, including our blood sugar levels.

The Stress Response and Blood Sugar Control

When we experience stress, whether physical or emotional, our bodies respond by releasing a hormone called cortisol. Cortisol helps to mobilize glucose (sugar) from the liver and muscles into the bloodstream, providing energy to deal with the stressor.

While this response can be helpful in the short-term, chronic or excessive stress can lead to chronically elevated cortisol levels and higher blood sugar levels over time. This can contribute to insulin resistance and an increased risk of type 2 diabetes.

Managing Stress to Support Healthy Blood Sugar Levels

Fortunately, there are many strategies for managing stress and supporting healthy blood sugar levels. Some effective stress-management strategies include:

1.Exercise: Regular physical activity has been shown to reduce stress and improve blood sugar control. Aim for at least 30 minutes of moderate-intensity exercise most days of the week.

2.Mindfulness meditation: Mindfulness meditation involves focusing on the present moment and letting go of distracting thoughts. It has been shown to reduce stress and improve blood sugar control. Consider taking a mindfulness meditation class or using an app to guide your practice.

3.Deep breathing: Deep breathing exercises can help to reduce stress and lower cortisol levels. Try taking deep, slow breaths in through your nose and out through your mouth for several minutes when you are feeling stressed.

4.Yoga: Yoga combines physical movement with breath work and meditation, making it an effective stress-management tool. Consider taking a yoga class or following along with a yoga video online.

5.Social support: Talking to friends and loved ones can help to reduce stress and improve mood. Consider joining a support group or talking to a counselor or therapist if you are struggling with chronic stress.

The Link between Sleep and Blood Sugar

Sleep plays an important role in regulating many hormones and processes in the body, including insulin sensitivity and glucose metabolism. During sleep, the body produces hormones that help to regulate blood sugar levels, including growth hormone, cortisol, and melatonin.

Inadequate sleep or poor sleep quality can disrupt the balance of these hormones, leading to insulin resistance, glucose intolerance, and increased levels of inflammation. This can increase the risk of developing type 2 diabetes and other health problems.

The Benefits of Sleep for Blood Sugar Management

Getting enough quality sleep offers a range of benefits for blood sugar management and overall health. These include:

1.Improved insulin sensitivity: Getting enough quality sleep helps to improve insulin sensitivity, allowing the body to use insulin more effectively to transport glucose into the cells.

2.Reduced inflammation: Sleep helps to reduce inflammation in the body, which is associated with insulin resistance and other health problems.

3.Lowered stress levels: Adequate sleep can help to reduce stress levels, which can improve blood sugar control and overall health.

4.Improved weight management: Sleep helps to regulate appetite hormones, reducing cravings and helping to maintain a healthy weight.

Strategies for Improving Sleep Quality

Improving sleep quality can help to support healthy blood sugar levels and overall health. Some strategies for improving sleep quality include:

1.Establishing a regular sleep schedule: Try to go to bed and wake up at the same time each day, even on weekends.

2.Creating a relaxing sleep environment: Make sure your bedroom is cool, quiet, and dark, and limit screen time before bed.

3.Practicing relaxation techniques: Meditation, deep breathing, and other relaxation techniques can help to reduce stress and improve sleep quality.

4.Avoiding caffeine and alcohol: Limit caffeine and alcohol intake, especially in the evening, as they can interfere with sleep quality.

5.Managing stress: Stress can interfere with sleep quality and blood sugar control. Strategies for managing stress include exercise, meditation, and counseling.

Conclusion

In conclusion, getting enough quality sleep is essential for blood sugar management and overall health. Adequate sleep helps to improve insulin sensitivity, reduce inflammation, lower stress levels, and support healthy weight management. By establishing a regular sleep schedule, creating a relaxing sleep environment, and practicing relaxation techniques, individuals can improve their sleep quality and support healthy blood sugar levels. In the following chapters, we will explore additional strategies for managing blood sugar levels, including nutrition and